CW00500363

The Sirtfood Diet Cookbook for Lunch Meals

50 simple and healthy recipes to give your lunch the right taste

Anne Patel

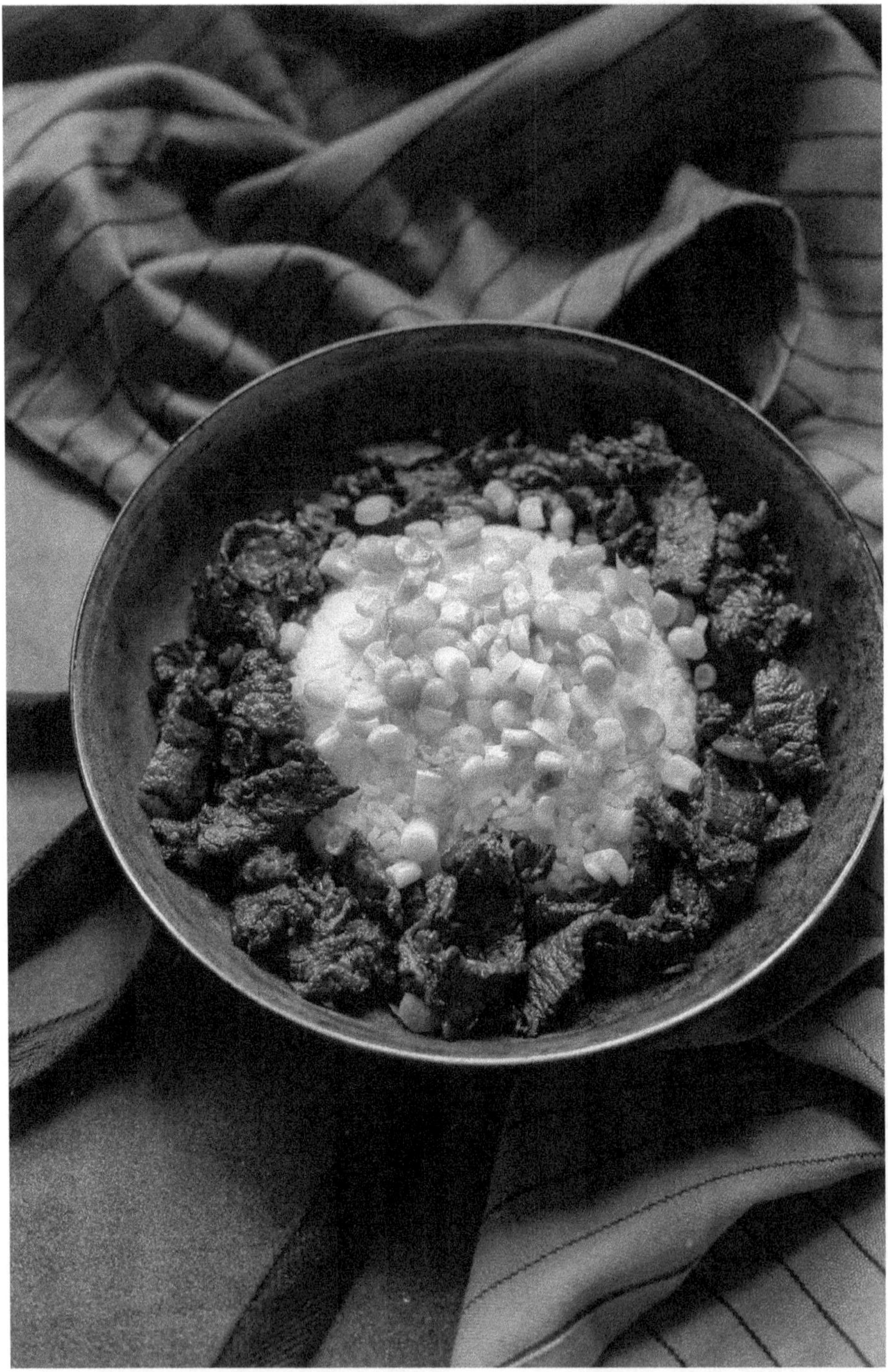

© Copyright 2021 - All rights reserved.

The content contained within this book may not be reproduced, duplicated or transmitted without direct written permission from the author or the publisher.

Under no circumstances will any blame or legal responsibility be held against the publisher, or author, for any damages, reparation, or monetary loss due to the information contained within this book. Either directly or indirectly.

Legal Notice:

This book is copyright protected. This book is only for personal use. You cannot amend, distribute, sell, use, quote or paraphrase any part, or the content within this book, without the consent of the author or publisher.

Disclaimer Notice:

Please note the information contained within this document is for educational and entertainment purposes only. All effort has been executed to present accurate, up to date, and reliable, complete information. No warranties of any kind are declared or implied. Readers acknowledge that the author is not engaging in the rendering of legal, financial, medical or professional advice. The content within this book has been derived from various sources. Please consult a licensed professional before attempting any techniques outlined in this book.

By reading this document, the reader agrees that under no circumstances is the author responsible for any losses, direct or indirect, which are incurred as a result of the use of information contained within this document, including, but not limited to, — errors, omissions, or inaccuracies.

Table of Contents

Chapter 1: What is the Sirtfood diet

The Sirtfood Diet was created by Masters in Nutritional Medicine, Aiden Goggins and Glen Matten.

Their goal initially was to find a healthier way for people to eat, but people started losing weight quickly when they tested their program. With all the people in the world following diets hoping to lose pounds, they thought it would be selfish not to disclose their innovative health plan.

The plan they developed focuses on combining certain foods eaten in order to maximize the supply of nutrition to our body. There is an initial phase in which calories are limited to give the body a period to recover and eliminate accumulated waste. A maintenance phase follows this first phase to accustom the metabolism to the new foods you are ingesting. Throughout all stages, you will incorporate potent green juices and well-structured, well-planned meals.

The diet focuses on so-called 'sirtfoods,' plant-based foods that are known to stimulate a gene called sirtuin in the human body. Sirtuins belong to an entire protein family, called SIRT1 to SIRT7, and each has specific health-related connections. These proteins help separate and safeguard our cells from inflammation and other damage resulting from everyday activities, helping to reduce our risk of developing major diseases, particularly those related to aging.

Studies have shown that people live longer and healthier lives when they eat diets rich in these foods that activate sirtuin, free from diabetes, heart disease, and even dementia. So this diet was designed to restore a healthy body situation, and one of the byproducts of a healthy body is also the loss of excess weight.

The diet Sirtfood is neither a miracle cure nor a week-long program designed to quickly lose weight before beach holidays. If you are only interested in losing a few pounds and then returning to your old habits, there are certainly plans and diets that are more suited to your needs.

The Sirtfood diet is a project born to help you for the rest of your life, using delicious foods, but that will also improve your health. If you switch from a standard American diet (SAD) to a sirtfood diet, you will lose all the weight your body does not need.

A healthy body does not store extra energy. It asks for what it needs and uses it effectively.
The diet isn't designed to encourage you to starve or deprive yourself. The fact is, foods that are deficient in nutrients are designer made to deprive you and, though the calories are there in plenty, your cells are still starved for the nutrition to help you thrive. The Sirtfood Diet is the opposite of deprivation and starvation. It is nourishment and balance.

Most people following the SAD may use 20 ingredients in a month, let alone enjoy the sheer volume of choice ingredients from the 120 options you will learn about here.

In recent decades, an alarming number of people have come to the conclusion that healthy food is boring, and plants or, more specifically, vegetables are terrible tasting. This is because the foods we've become dependent on – packed with sugar, salt, and unhealthy fats – have chemically altered our connection to food. Our brains are essentially lying to us, and our taste buds have been compromised.

This is one of the reasons the week-long reset is so important. After this first week, you will be able to taste food differently. The more you expose yourself to the recommended plant-based foods, the more pleasure you get out of them.

Sirtuins are critical for our health, regulating many essential biological functions, including our metabolism, which, I'm sure you know, is very closely connected to our weight. It's also a key figure in determining our body composition, such as how much muscle we build and how much fat we retain.

Sirtuin genes regulate all this and more. They're also integral in the process of aging and disease.

If we can turn these genes on, we'll be able to protect our cells and enjoy better health for longer life. Eating sirtfoods is the most effective way to accomplish this goal.

Sirtfoods are all plant-based, and they have many more benefits, in addition to being sirtuin activators.

Our bodies require energy to operate, and the majority of this fuel comes from three primary macronutrients: carbohydrates, fats, and proteins. These macros largely control our metabolic system and regulate how the calories we consume get processed by our bodies. This is why most diets focus exclusively on micronutrition and require you to calculate calories.

Our bodies need more than just energy to survive than thriving, however, which is why micronutrients are so important. They don't impact our weight as obviously as macros, but they are our health foundations.

Micronutrients, such as vitamins, minerals, fiber, antioxidants, and phytonutrients, are supposed to be consumed along with our calories. Unfortunately, in the Standard American Diet (SAD), they're in very limited supply.

When your diet is primarily made up of large quantities of red meat and processed meats, pre-packaged foods, vegetable oils, refined grains and a lot of sugar, you will have an almost total lack of micronutrition.

Plant foods offer the most micronutrients per calorie consumed. Every edible plant has a unique nutritional profile, protecting you from an innumerable variety of illnesses.

Sirtfoods, and other plant-based sources of nutrition, give your body what it needs to stay young and disease-free, and, as a bonus, this will help you remain at an ideal weight.

The original Sirtfood Diet encourages you to commit to a one week reset phase and then a 2-week maintenance phase where you rely heavily on the Sirtfood green juice for a significant dose of nutrition along with meals rich in sirtfoods. Once the phases are complete, to retain your health for the rest of your life, you will need to continue incorporating these sirtfoods into your daily meals.

The Sirtfood Diet is not a miracle cure, but if you stick to these recipes, you'll not just impress your taste buds, but you'll also enhance nearly every aspect of your health. To get safe, you don't have to count calories or starve yourself, the youthful body you've always wanted.

Sirtfood Diet Phases

Every newbie needs to understand that the sirtfood diet does not start with a single list of ingredients in your hands. Its implementation and adaptation are more than mere selective grocery shopping. Every diet can only work effectively when we allow our body to embrace the sudden shift and change in food intake. Similarly, the sirtfood diet also comes with two phases of adaptation. If a dieter successfully goes through these phases, he can continue with the sirtfood diet easily. There are mainly two phases of this diet, which are then succeeded by a third phase in which you can decide how you want to continue the diet.

Phase One

The first seven days of this diet plan are characterized as Phase One. In this phase, a dieter must focus on calorie restriction and the intake of green juices. These seven days are crucial to initiate your weight loss and usually help to lose up to seven pounds if the diet is followed properly. If you find yourself achieving this target, that means that you are on the right track.

In the first three days of the first phase, a dieter must restrict this caloric intake to 1,000 calories only. While doing so, the dieter must also have green juice throughout the day, probably three times a day. Try to drink green juice per meal. The recipes given in the book are perfect for selecting from.

Many meal options can keep your caloric intake in checks, such as buckwheat noodles, seared tofu, some shrimp stir fry, or sirtfood omelet.

Once the first three days of this diet has passed, you can increase your caloric intake to 1,500 calories per day. In these next four days, you can reduce the green juices to two times per side. And pair the juices with more Sirtuin-rich food in every meal.

Phase Two

After the first week of the sirtfood diet, then starts phase two. This phase is more about the maintenance of the diet, as the first week enables the body to embrace the change and start working according to the new diet. This phase enables the body to continue working towards the weight loss objective slowly and steadily. Therefore, the duration of this phase is almost two weeks.

So how is this phase different from phase one? In this phase, there is no restriction on the caloric intake, as long as the food is rich in sirtuins and you are taking it three times a day, it is good to go. Instead of having the green juice two or three times a day, the dieter can have juice one time a day, and that will be enough to achieve steady weight loss. You can have the juice after any meal, in the morning or in the evening.

After the Diet Phase

With the end of phase two comes the time, which is most crucial, and that is the after-diet phase. If your weight loss target has not been reached by the end of step two, then you can restart the phases all over again. Or even when you have achieved the goals but still want to lose more weight, then you can again give it a try.

Instead of following phases one and two over and over again, you can also continue having good quality sirtfood meals in this after-diet phase. Simply continue the eating practices of phase two, have a diet rich in sirtuin and do have green juices whenever possible. The diet is mainly divided into two phases: the first lasts one week, and the other lasts 14 days.

The best 20 sirt foods

All these foods include high quantities of plant compounds called polyphenols, which can be thought to modify the sirtuin enzymes, therefore, excite their super-healthy added benefits.

Top 20 sirtfoods

1. Arugula (Rocket)
2. Buckwheat
3. Capers
4. Celery
5. Chilis
6. Cocoa
7. Coffee
8. Extra Virgin Olive Oil
9. Garlic
10. Green Tea (especially Matcha)
11. Kale
12. Medjool Dates
13. Parsley
14. Red Endive
15. Red Onions
16. Red Wine
17. Soy
18. Strawberries
19. Turmeric
20. Walnuts

What Is So Great About Sirtuins?

There are seven types of Sirtuins named from **SIRT1** to **SIRT7**. Although our understanding of the exact functions of all the Sirtuins is minimal, studies show that activating them can have the following benefits:

Switching on fat burning and protection from weight gain: Sirtuins do this by increasing the mitochondrion's functionality (which is involved in the production of energy) and sparking a change in your metabolism to break down more fat cells.

Improving Memory by protecting neurons from damage. Sirtuins also boost learning skills and memory through the enhancement of synaptic plasticity. Synaptic plasticity refers to synapses' capacity to weaken or strengthen with time due to decreased or increased activity. This is important because memories are represented by different interconnected networks of synapses in the brain, and synaptic plasticity is an important neurochemical foundation of memory and learning.

Slowing down the Ageing Process: Sirtuins act as cell guarding enzymes. Thus, they protect the cells and slow down their aging process.

Repairing cells: The Sirtuins repair cells damaged by re-activating cell functionality.

Protection against diabetes: this happens through prevention against insulin resistance. Sirtuins do this by controlling blood sugar levels because this diet calls for moderate consumption of carbohydrates. These foods cause increases in blood sugar levels; hence the need to release insulin, and as the blood sugar levels increase greatly, there is a need to produce more insulin.

Over time, cells become resistant to insulin, hence producing more insulin and leading to insulin resistance.

Fighting Cancers: The chemicals working as sirtuin activators affect the function of sirtuin in different cells, i.e. by switching it on when in normal cells and shutting it down in cancerous cells. This encourages the death of cancerous cells.

Fighting inflammation: Sirtuins have a powerful antioxidant effect that has the power to reduce oxidative stress. This has positive effects on heart health and cardiovascular protection.

Chapter 2: How do the Sirtfood Diet Works?

The basis of the sirtuin diet can be explained in simple terms or in complex ways. However, it's important to understand how and why it works so that you can appreciate the value of what you are doing. It is important to also know why these sirtuin rich foods help to help you maintain fidelity to your diet plan. Otherwise, you may throw something in your meal with less nutrition that would defeat the purpose of planning for one rich in sirtuins. Most importantly, this is not a dietary fad, and as you will see, there is much wisdom contained in how humans have used natural foods, even for medicinal purposes, over thousands of years.

To understand how the Sirtfood diet works and why these particular foods are necessary, we're going to look at their role in the human body.

Sirtuin activity was first researched in yeast, where a mutation caused an extension in the yeast's lifespan. Sirtuins were also shown to slow aging in laboratory mice, fruit flies, and nematodes. As research on Sirtuins proved to transfer to mammals, they were examined for their use in diet and slowing the aging process. The sirtuins in humans are different in typing, but they essentially work in the same ways and reasons.

The Sirtuin family is made up of seven "members." It is believed that sirtuins play a big role in regulating certain functions of cells, including proliferation, reproduction and growth of cells), apoptosis death of cells). They promote survival and resist stress to increase longevity.

They are also seen to block neurodegeneration loss or function of the nerve cells in the brain). They conduct their housekeeping functions by cleaning out toxic proteins and supporting the brain's ability to change and adapt to different conditions or to recuperate i.e., brain plasticity). They also help minimize chronic inflammation as part of this and decrease anything called oxidative stress. Oxidative stress is when there are so many free radicals present in the body that are cell-damaging, and by fighting them with antioxidants, the body can not keep up. These factors are related to age-related illness and weight as well, which again brings us back to a discussion of how they actually work.

You will see labels in Sirtuins that start with "SIR," which represents "Silence Information Regulator" genes. They do exactly that, silence or regulate, as part of their functions. Humans work with the seven sirtuins: SIRT1, SIRT2, SIRT3, SIRT4, SIRT 5, SIRT6 and SIRT7. Each of these types is responsible for different areas of protecting cells. They work by either stimulating or turning on certain gene expressions or by reducing and turning off other gene expressions. This essentially means that they can influence genes to do more or less of something, most of which they are already programmed to do.

Through enzyme reactions, each of the SIRT types affects different areas of cells responsible for the metabolic processes that help maintain life. This is also related to what organs and functions they will affect.

For example, the SIRT6 causes and expression of genes in humans that affect skeletal muscle, fat tissue, brain, and heart. SIRT 3 would cause an expression of genes that affect the kidneys, liver, brain and heart.

If we tie these concepts together, you can see that the Sirtuin proteins can change the expression of genes, and in the case of the Sirtfood diet, we care about how sirtuins can turn off those genes that are responsible for speeding up aging and for weight management.

The other aspect to this conversation of sirtuins is the function and the power of calorie restriction on the human body. Calorie restriction is simply eating fewer calories. This, coupled with exercise and reducing stress, is usually a combination for weight loss. Calorie restriction has also proven across much research in animals and humans to increase one's lifespan.

We can look further at the role of sirtuins with calorie restriction and using the SIRT3 protein, which has a role in metabolism and aging. Amongst all of the effects of the protein on gene expression, such as preventing cells from dying, reducing tumors from growing, etc.), we want to understand the effects of SIRT3 on weight for this book's purpose.

As we stated earlier, the SIRT3 has high expression in those metabolically active tissues, and its ability to express itself increases with caloric restriction, fasting, and exercise. On the contrary, it will express itself less when the body has high fat, high calorie-riddled diet.

The last few highlights of sirtuins are their role in regulating telomeres and reducing inflammation, which also helps with staving off disease and aging. Telomeres are sequences of proteins at the ends of chromosomes. When cells divide, these get shorter. As we age, they get shorter, and other stressors to the body also will contribute to this. Maintaining these longer telomeres is the key to slower aging. In addition, proper diet, along with exercise and other variables, can lengthen telomeres. SIRT6 is one of the sirtuins that, if activated, can help with DNA damage, inflammation and oxidative stress. SIRT1 also helps with inflammatory response cycles that are related to many age-related diseases.

Calories restriction can extend life to some degree. Since this and fasting are a stressor, these factors will stimulate the SIRT3 proteins to kick in and protect the body from the stressors and excess free radicals. Again, the telomere length is affected as well.

Having laid this all out before you, you should appreciate how and why these miraculous compounds work in your favor, keep you youthful, healthy, and lean If they are working hard for you, don't you feel that you should do something too?

50 Essential Lunch Recipes

1. Sticky Chicken Watermelon Noodle Salad

Preparation Time: 20 minutes
Cooking time: 40 minutes
Servings: 2

Ingredients
2 pieces of skinny rice noodles
1/2 tbsp. sesame oil
2 cups watermelon
Head of bib lettuce
Half of a lot of scallions
Half of a lot of fresh cilantro
2 skinless, boneless chicken breasts
1/2 tbsp. Chinese five-spice
1 tbsp. extra virgin olive oil
Two tbsp. sweet skillet (I utilized a mixture of maple syrup using a dash of tabasco)
1 tbsp. sesame seeds
A couple of cashews - smashed Dressing - could be made daily or 2 until 1 tbsp. low-salt soy sauce 1 teaspoon sesame oil
1 tbsp. peanut butter
Half of a refreshing red chili
Half of a couple of chives
Half of a couple of cilantros
1 lime - juiced

1 small spoonful of garlic

Directions:

1. In a bowl, then completely substituting the noodles in boiling drinking water. They are going to be soon spread out in 2 minutes.

2. On a big sheet of parchment paper, throw the chicken with pepper, salt, and the five-spice.

3. Twist over the paper subsequently flattens the chicken using a rolling pin.

4. Place into the large skillet with 1 tbsp. of olive oil, turning 3 or 4 minutes, until well charred and cooked through.

5. Using 1 tbsp to remove the noodles and toss. Sesame oil on a large serving platter.

6. Place 50% the noodles into the moderate skillet, frequently stirring until crispy and nice.

7. Remove the watermelon skin, then slice the flesh to inconsistent balls, and then move to plate.

8. Wash the lettuces and cut into small wedges and half of a whole lot of leafy greens and scatter on the dish.

9. Place another 1 / 2 the cilantro pack, the soy sauce, coriander, chives, peanut butter, 1 teaspoon of sesame oil, a dab of water, and the lime juice in a bowl, then mix till smooth.

10. set the chicken back to heat, garnish with all the sweet sauce (or my walnut syrup mixture) and toss with the sesame seeds.

11. Pour the dressing on the salad toss gently with clean fingers until well coated, then add crispy noodles and then smashed cashews.

12. Mix chicken pieces and add them to the salad.

Nutrition: Calories: 694 Carbohydrates: 0 Fat: 33g Protein: 0

2. Fruity Curry Chicken Salad

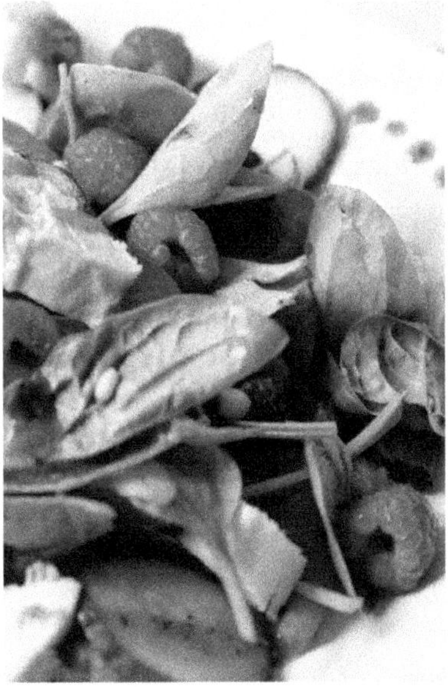

Preparation Time: 20 minutes

Cooking time: 10 minutes

Servings: 2

Ingredients

Original recipe yields 8 servings

Fixing checklist

4 skinless, boneless chicken pliers - cooked and diced

1 tsp celery, diced

4 green onions, sliced

1 golden delicious apple peeled, cored, and diced

1/3 cup golden raisins

1/3 cup seedless green grapes, halved

1/2 cup sliced toasted pecans

1/8 Teaspoon ground black pepper

1/2 tsp curry powder

3/4 cup light mayonnaise

Directions:

1. In a big bowl, combine the chicken, onion, celery, apple, celery, celery, pecans, pepper, curry powder, and carrot. Mix altogether. Enjoy!

Nutrition: Fat; 44 milligrams Cholesterol: 188 milligrams Sodium. 12.3 g Carbohydrates: 15.1 gram of Protein; full nutrition

3. Zuppa Toscana

Preparation Time: 25 minutes
Cooking time: 60 minutes
Servings: 2

Ingredients
1 lb. ground Italian sausage
1 1/4 tsp of crushed of red pepper flakes
4 pieces bacon, cut into ½ inch bits
1 big onion, diced
1 tbsp. minced garlic
5 (13.75 oz.) can chicken broth
6 celery, thinly chopped
1 cup thick cream
1/4 bunch fresh spinach, tough stems removed

Directions:
1. Cook that the Italian sausage and red pepper flakes in a pot on medium-high heat until crumbly, browned, with no longer pink, 10 to 15minutes. Drain and put aside.

2. Cook the bacon at the exact Dutch oven over moderate heat until crispy, about 10 minutes. Drain, leaving a couple of tablespoons of drippings together with all the bacon at the bottom of the toaster. Stir in the garlic and onions cook until onions are tender and translucent, about five minutes.

3. Pour the chicken broth to the pot with the onion and bacon mix; contribute to a boil on high temperature. Add the berries and boil until fork-tender, about 20 minutes.

4. Reduce heat to moderate and stir in the cream and the cooked sausage – heat throughout. Mix the lettuce to the soup before serving.

Nutrition: Carbohydrates; 32.6 g Fat; 45.8 g Carbs; 19.8 g Protein; 99 Milligrams Cholesterol: 2386

4. Country Chicken Breasts

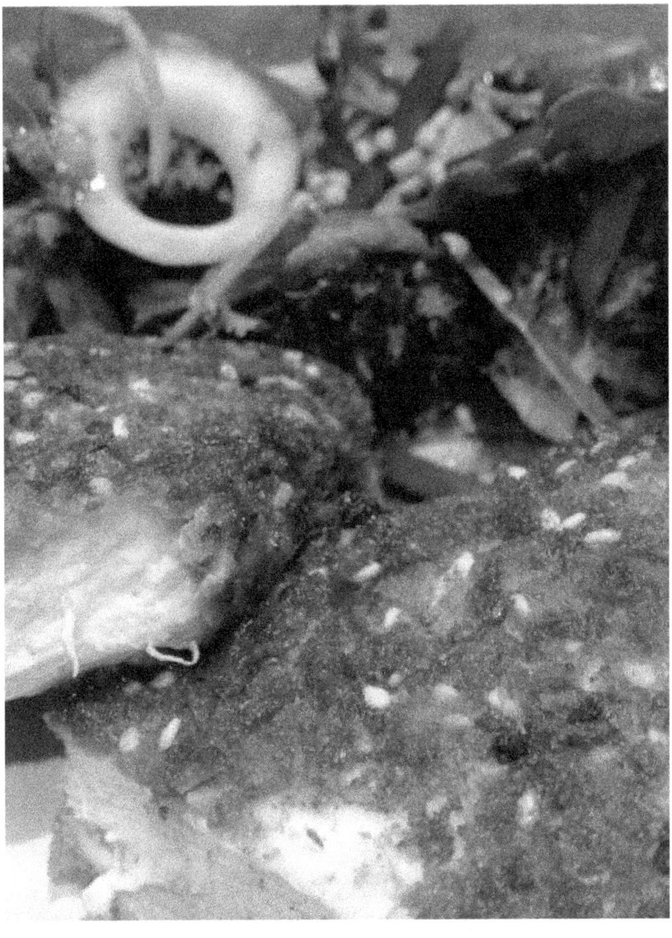

Preparation Time: 10 minutes

Cooking Time: 45 minutes

Servings: 2

Ingredients:

2 medium green apples, diced
1 small red onion, finely diced
1 small green bell pepper, chopped
3 cloves garlic, minced
2 tablespoons dried currants
1 tablespoon curry powder
1 teaspoon turmeric
1 teaspoon ground ginger
¼ teaspoon chili pepper flakes
1 can (14 ½ ounce) diced tomatoes
6 skinless, boneless chicken breasts, halved
½ cup chicken broth
1 cup long-grain white rice
1-pound large raw shrimp, shelled and deveined
Salt and pepper to taste
Chopped parsley
1/3 cup slivered almonds

Directions:

1. Rinse chicken, pat dry and set aside.

2. In a large crockpot, combine apples, onion, bell pepper, garlic, currants, curry powder, turmeric, ginger, and chili pepper flakes. Stir in tomatoes.

3. Arrange chicken, overlapping pieces slightly, on top of tomato mixture.

4. Pour in broth and do not mix or stir.

5. Cover and cook at for 6 – 7 hours on low.

6. Preheat oven to 200 degrees F.

7. Carefully transfer chicken to an oven-safe plate, cover lightly, and keep warm in the oven.

8. Stir rice into remaining liquid. Increase the heat setting of the cooker to high; cover and cook, stirring once or twice, until rice is almost tender to bite, 30 to 35 minutes. Stir in the shrimp, cover and cook until the middle of the shrimp is opaque, about 10 more minutes.

9. Meanwhile, toast almonds in a small pan over medium heat until golden brown, 5 - 8 minutes, stirring occasionally. Set aside.

10. Mound in a warm serving dish and arrange chicken on top. Sprinkle with parsley and almonds.

Nutrition: Calories: 155 Carbs: 13.9g Protein: 17.4g Fat: 3.8g

5. Apples and Cabbage Mix

Preparation Time: 5 minutes
Cooking Time: 0 minutes
Servings: 4

Ingredients:

2 cored and cubed green apples
2tbsps. Balsamic vinegar
½ tsp. caraway seeds
2tbsps. olive oil
Black pepper
1 shredded red cabbage head

Directions:

1. Mix the cabbage with the apples and the other ingredients in a dish, toss and serve.

Nutrition: Calories: 165 Fat: 7.4 g Carbs: 26 g Protein: 2.6 g Sugars: 2.6 g Sodium: 19 mg

6. Rosemary Endives

Preparation Time: 10 minutes
Cooking Time: 45 minutes
Servings: 2

Ingredients:

2tbsps. olive oil

1 tsp. dried rosemary

2 halved endives

¼ tsp. black pepper

½ tsp. turmeric powder

Directions:

1. In a baking pan, combine the endives with the oil and the other ingredients, toss gently, introduce in the oven and bake at 400 oF for 20 minutes.

2. Divide between plates and serve.

Nutrition: Calories: 66 Fat: 7.1 g Carbs: 1.2 g Protein: 0.3 g Sugars: 1.3 g Sodium: 113 mg

7. Kale Sauté

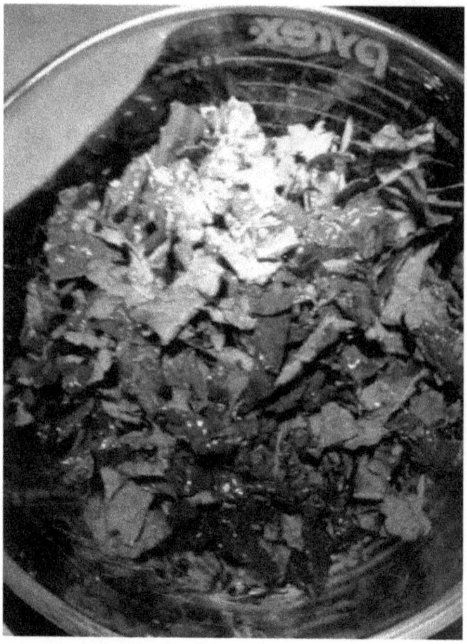

Preparation Time: 10 minutes

Cooking Time: 35 minutes

Servings: 2

Ingredients:

1 chopped red onion

3tbsps. coconut aminos

2tbsps. olive oil

1 lb. torn kale

1 tbsp. chopped cilantro

1 tbsp. lime juice

2 minced garlic cloves

Directions:

1. Heat a pan over medium heat with the olive oil, add the onion and the garlic and sauté for 5 minutes.

2. Add the kale and the other ingredients, toss, cook over medium heat for 10 minutes, divide between plates and serve.

Nutrition: Calories: 200 Fat: 7.1 g Carbs: 6.4 g Protein: 6 g Sugars: 1.6 g Sodium: 183 mg

8. Roasted Beets

Preparation Time: 10 minutes
Cooking Time: 40 minutes
Servings: 2

Ingredients:

2 minced garlic cloves
¼ tsp. black pepper
4 peeled and sliced beets
¼ c. chopped walnuts
2tbsps. olive oil
¼ c. chopped parsley

Directions:

1. In a baking dish, combine the beets with the oil and the other ingredients, toss to coat, introduce in the oven at 420 oF, and bake for 30 minutes.

2. Divide between plates and serve.

Nutrition: Calories: 156 Fat: 11.8 g Carbs: 11.5 g Protein: 3.8 g Sugars: 8 g Sodium: 670 mg

9. Minty Tomatoes and Corn

Preparation Time: 10 minutes

Cooking Time: 65 minutes

Servings: 2

Ingredients:

2 c. corn

1 tbsp. rosemary vinegar

2tbsps. chopped minutest

1 lb. sliced tomatoes

¼ tsp. black pepper

2tbsps. olive oil

Directions:

1. In a salad bowl, combine the tomatoes with the corn and the other ingredients, toss and serve.

Nutrition: Calories: 230 Fat: 7.2 g Carbs: 11.6 g Protein: 4 g Sugars: 1 g Sodium: 53 mg

10. Pesto Green Beans

Preparation Time: 10 minutes
Cooking Time: 55 minutes
Servings: 2

Ingredients:

2tbsps. olive oil

2 tsps. Sweet paprika

Juice of 1 lemon

2tbsps. basil pesto

1 lb. trimmed and halved green beans

¼ tsp. black pepper

1 sliced red onion

Directions:

1. Over medium-high pressure, heat a pan with the oil, add the onion, stir and sauté for 5 minutes.

2. Add the beans and the rest of the ingredients, toss, cook over medium heat for 10 minutes, divide between plates and serve.

Nutrition: Calories: 280 Fat: 10 g Carbs: 13.9 g Protein: 4.7 g Sugars: 0.8 g Sodium: 138 mg

11. Scallops and Sweet Potatoes

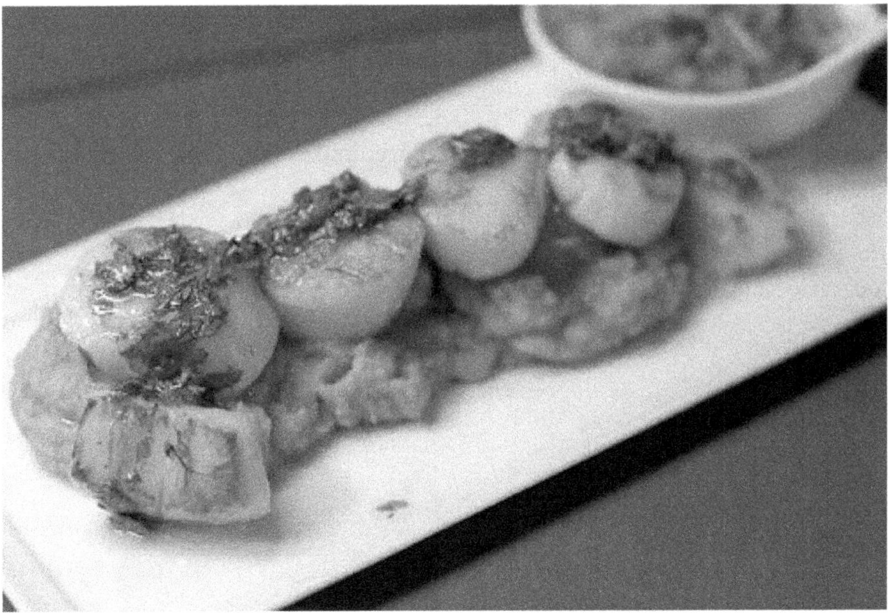

Preparation Time: 5 minutes

Cooking Time: 22 minutes

Servings: 4

Ingredients:

1-pound scallops

½ teaspoon rosemary, dried

½ teaspoon oregano, dried

2 tablespoons avocado oil

1 yellow onion, chopped

2 sweet potatoes, peeled and cubed

½ cup chicken stock

1 tablespoon cilantro, chopped

Directions:

1. Heat a pan with the oil on medium heat, add the onion and sauté for 2 minutes.

2. Add the sweet potatoes and the stock, toss and cook for 10 minutes more.

3. Add the scallops and the remaining ingredients, toss, cook for another10 minutes, divide everything into bowls and serve.

Nutrition: Calories 211 Fat 2 Fiber 4.1 Carbs 26.9 Protein 20.7

12. Citrus Salmon

Preparation Time: 10 minutes
Cooking Time: 45 minutes
Servings: 2

Ingredients:

1 ½ lb. salmon fillet with skin on
Salt and pepper to taste
1 medium red onion, chopped
2 tablespoons parsley, chopped
2 teaspoons lemon rind, grated
2 teaspoons orange rind, grated
2 tablespoons extra virgin olive oil
1 lemon, sliced thinly
1 orange, sliced thinly
1 cup vegetable broth

Directions:

1. Line your crockpot with parchment paper and top with the lemon slices.

2. Season salmon with salt and pepper and place it on top of lemon.

3. Cover the fish with the onion, parsley and grated citrus rinds and oil over fish. Top with orange slices, reserving a few for garnish.

4. Pour broth around, but not directly overtop, your salmon.

5. Cover and cook for 2 hours under low pressure.

6. Preheat oven to 400 degrees F.

7. When salmon is opaque and flaky, remove from the crockpot carefully using the parchment paper and transfer to a baking sheet. Place in the oven for 5 – 8 minutes to allow the salmon to brown on top.

8. Serve garnished with orange and lemon slices.

Nutrition: Calories 294 Fat 3 Fiber 8 Carbs 49 Protein 21

13. Sage Carrots

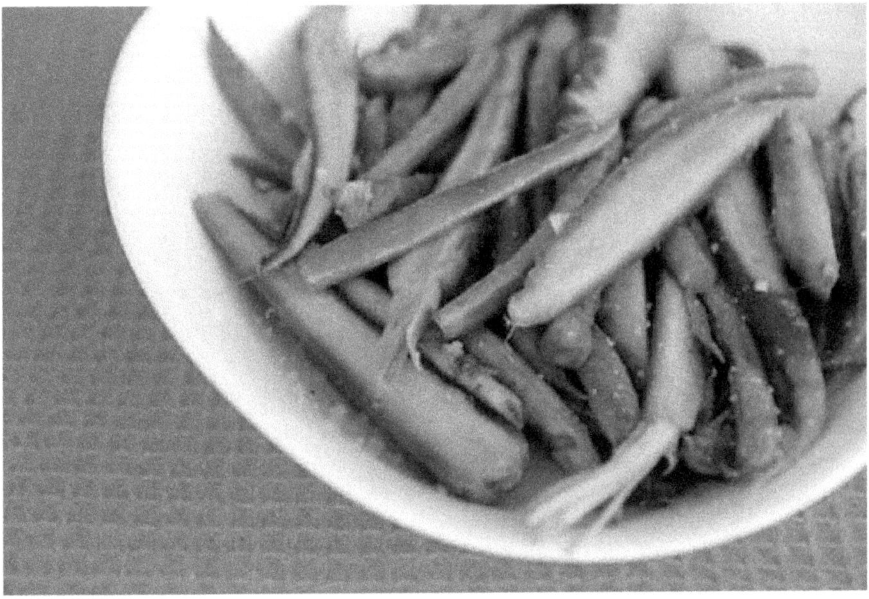

Preparation Time: 10 minutes

Cooking Time: 25 minutes

Servings: 2

Ingredients:

2 tsps. Sweet paprika

1 tbsp. chopped sage

2tbsps. olive oil

1 lb. peeled and roughly cubed carrots

¼ tsp. black pepper

1 chopped red onion

Directions:

1. In a baking pan, combine the carrots with the oil and the other ingredients, toss and bake at 380 oF for 30 minutes.

2. Divide between plates and serve.

Nutrition: Calories: 200 Fat: 8.7 g Carbs: 7.9 g Protein: 4 g Sugars: 19 g Sodium: 268 mg

14. Moong Dahl

Preparation Time: 10 minutes
Cooking Time: 10 minutes
Servings: 4-6

Ingredients:

300g/10oz split mung beans (moong dahl)
Preferably soaked for a few hours
600ml/1pt of water
2 tbsp./30g olive oil, butter or ghee
1 red onion, finely chopped
1-2 tsp coriander seeds
1-2 tsp cumin seeds
2-4 tsp fresh ginger, chopped
1-2 tsp turmeric
¼ tsp of cayenne pepper – more if you want it spicy
Salt & black pepper to taste

Directions:

1. First drain and rinse the split mung beans. Put them in a saucepan, then cover them with water. Bring to the boil and skim off any foam that arises. Turn down the heat, cover and simmer.

2. Meanwhile, in a pan, heat the oil and fry the onion until the onion becomes soft.

3. In a heavy-bottomed pan, fry the coriander and cumin seeds dryly. Fry until they start to pop. Grind them in a pestle and mortar.

4. Add the ground spices to the onions and also add ginger, turmeric and cayenne pepper. Cook for a few minutes.

5. Once the mung beans are almost done, add the onion and spice mix to them. With salt and pepper, season and cook for another 10 minutes.

Nutrition: Calories 347 Protein 25.73 Fiber 18.06

15. Macaroni & Cheese with Broccoli

Preparation Time: 10 minutes
Cooking Time: 6 minutes
Servings: 6

Ingredients:
3cups whole-wheat macaroni, uncooked 1large fresh broccoli crown, chopped
¼cup flour
2.5cups milk, divided
1½cups shredded extra-sharp cheddar cheese 2teaspoons Dijon mustard
¼teaspoon garlic powder
¾teaspoon paprika
¼teaspoon salt
2teaspoons extra virgin olive oil
Crumb topping
Cooking spray
3tablespoons dry breadcrumbs
¾teaspoon salt
¼teaspoon white pepper

Directions:
1. Preheat oven to 400° F. Coat a 2-quart baking dish with cooking spray. Bring to a boil a large pot of salted water.

2. When water boils cook macaroni 4 minutes. Add the raw fresh broccoli. Continue to cook until the pasta is slightly undercooked, for 2 minutes longer; the broccoli should be bright green and tender.

3. Meanwhile, prepare the sauce with cheese. Heat 2 cups of milk over medium-high heat in a medium saucepan, stirring frequently until heated. In a medium bowl, whisk together the remaining 1⁄2 cup of cold milk, flour, Dijon mustard, 3⁄4 teaspoon salt and white pepper until fully smooth. In the steaming milk, mix the flour mixture and bring to a simmer, whisking frequently until smooth and thickened.

4. In the pasta, stir the cheese sauce. Move the pasta mixture into the baking dish that has been prepared. In a small cup, whisk together the breadcrumbs, paprika, 1⁄4 teaspoon of salt, and garlic powder. Sprinkle with olive oil and stir until completely mixed. The crumbs are poured over the pasta and moved to the oven.

Nutrition: Energy (calories):397; Fat:7.1g; Carbohydrates:59.9g; Protein:20.5g

16. Glazed Tofu with Vegetables and Buckwheat

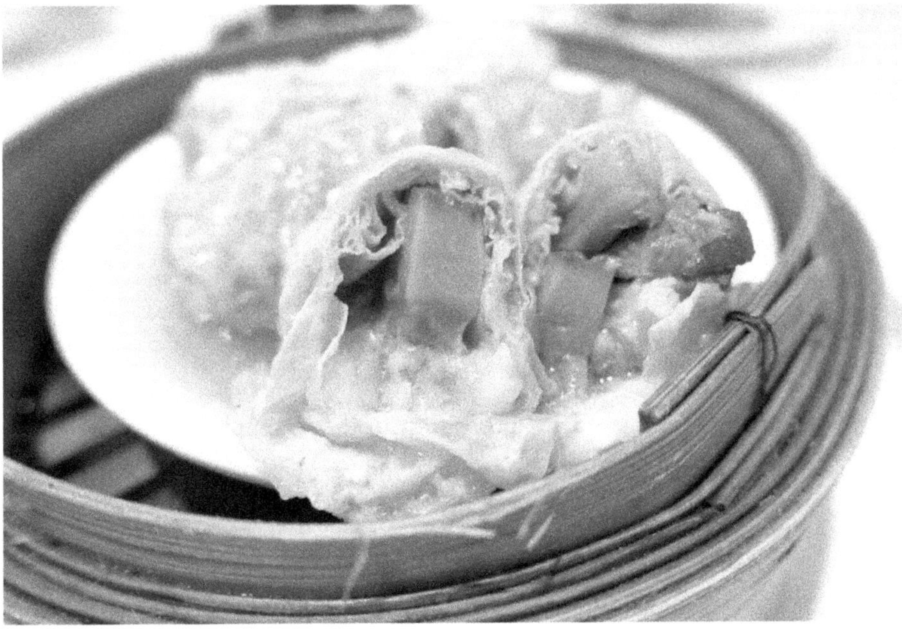

Preparation Time: 10 minutes.

Cooking Time: 20 minutes.

Servings: 1.

Ingredients:

150g tofu

1 tablespoon of mirin

20g Miso paste

40g green celery stalk

35g red onion

120g courgetti

1 small Thai chili

1 garlic clove

1 small piece of ginger

50g kale

2 teaspoons sesame seeds

35g buckwheat

1 teaspoon turmeric

2 teaspoons of extra virgin olive oil

1 teaspoon soy sauce or tamari

Directions:

1. Preheat oven to 400 °.

2. In the meantime, mix mirin and miso. Cut the tofu in half lengthwise and divide into two triangles. Briefly marinate the tofu with the mirin/miso paste while preparing the other ingredients.

3. Cut the celery stalks into thin slices, the zucchini into thick rings and the onion into thin rings. Finely chop garlic, ginger and chili. Coarsely chop the kale and stew or blanch briefly.

4. Place the marinated tofu in a small casserole dish, sprinkle with the sesame seeds and bake in the oven for approx. 15 minutes until the marinade has caramelized slightly.

5. In the meantime, cook the buckwheat according to the package instructions and add turmeric to the water.

6. Meanwhile, in a coated pan, heat the olive oil and add the celery, onion, courgette, chili, ginger and garlic—cook over high heat for one to two minutes, then two to three minutes at low temperature. Add a little water as required.

7. Serve the glazed tofu with vegetables and buckwheat.

Nutrition: Calories: 454 Fat: 24.2g. Carbs: 46.5g. Protein: 17.3g.

17. Tofu with Cauliflower

Preparation Time: 10 minutes.

Cooking Time: 50 minutes.

Servings: 1

Ingredients:

60g red pepper, seeded

1 Thai chili, cut in two halves, seeded

2 cloves of garlic

1 teaspoon of olive oil

1 pinch of cumin

1 pinch of coriander

Juice of a 1/4 lemon

200g tofu

200g cauliflower, roughly chopped

40g red onions, finely chopped

1 teaspoon finely chopped ginger

2 teaspoons turmeric

30g dried tomatoes, finely chopped

20g parsley, chopped

Directions:

1. Preheat oven to 400 °. Slice the peppers and put them in an ovenproof dish with chili and garlic. Pour some olive oil over it, add the dried herbs and put it in the oven Until the softness of the peppers is (about 20 minutes). Let it cool down, put the peppers together with the lemon juice in a blender and work it into a soft mass.

2. Cut the tofu in half and divide the halves into triangles. Place the tofu in a small casserole dish, cover with the paprika mixture and place in the oven for about 20 minutes.

3. Chop the cauliflower until the pieces are smaller than a grain of rice.

4. Then, in a small saucepan, heat the garlic, onions, chili and ginger with olive oil until they become transparent. Add turmeric and cauliflower, mix well and heat again. Remove from heat and add parsley and tomatoes, mix well. Serve with the tofu in the sauce.

Nutrition: Calories: 197.3 Fat: 9.4 g. Carbohydrate: 19.3 g Protein: 13.5 g

18. Filled Pita Pockets

Preparation Time: 20 minutes.
Cooking Time: 0 minutes.
Servings: 1

Ingredients:

You need whole-grain pita bags.
For a filling with meat:
80g roasted turkey breast
25g rocket salad, finely chopped
20g cheese, grated
35g cucumbers, small diced
30g red onions, finely diced
15g walnuts, chopped
Dressing of 1 tablespoon balsamic vinegar and 1 tablespoon extra-virgin olive oil

For a vegan filling:
3 tablespoons hummus
35g cucumbers, small diced
30g red onions, finely diced
25g rocket salad, finely chopped
15g walnuts, chopped
Dressing of 1 tablespoon of extra virgin olive oil and some lemon juice

Directions:

In both variations, mix all the ingredients, fill the pita pockets with them and marinate them with the dressing.

Nutrition: Calories: 120 Fat: 1g. Carbohydrate: 23g. Protein: 21g

19. Lima Bean Dip with Celery and Crackers

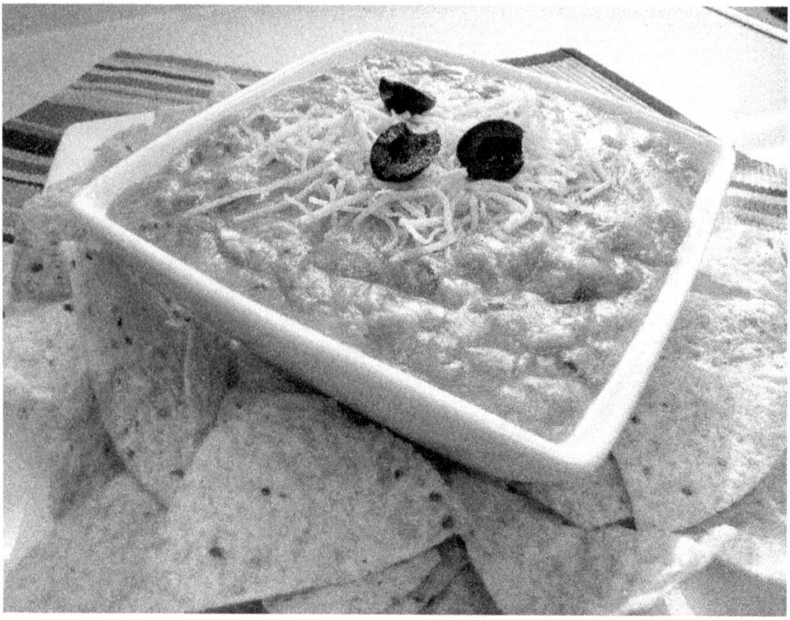

Preparation Time: 10 minutes.

Cooking Time: 0 minutes.

Servings: 2

Ingredients:

400g Lima beans or white beans from the tin

3 tablespoons of olive oil

Juice and zest of half an untreated lemon

4 spring onions, cut into fine rings

1 garlic clove, pressed

1/4 Thai chili, chopped

Directions:

1. Drain the beans. Then mix all ingredients with a potato masher to a mass.

2. Serve with green celery sticks and crackers.

Nutrition: Calories: 88 Fat: 0.7g. Carbohydrates: 15.7g. Protein: 5.3g.

20. Spinach and Eggplant Casserole

Preparation Time: 15 minutes.
Cooking Time: 55 minutes.
Servings: 3

Ingredients:

Eggplant
Onion slices
A spoon of olive oil
450 g spinach (fresh)
Tomato
Egg
60 ml of almond milk
1 teaspoon lemon juice
Almond flour

Directions:

1. Preheat the oven to 200 ° C.

2. Using olive oil to clean the eggplant and onions and fry them in the pan.

3. Place spinach in a large pot, heat over medium heat, then drain the colander.

4. Put the vegetables in a frying pan: first eggplant, then spinach, then onions and tomatoes. Repeat again

5. Beat eggs with almond milk, lemon juice, salt and pepper, then pour them on the vegetables.

6. Sprinkle almond flour on a plate and bake for about 30 to 40 minutes.

Nutrition: Calories: 139.9 Fat: 6.5 g. Carbohydrate: 21.5 g. Protein: 10.3 g.

21. Ancient Mediterranean Pizza

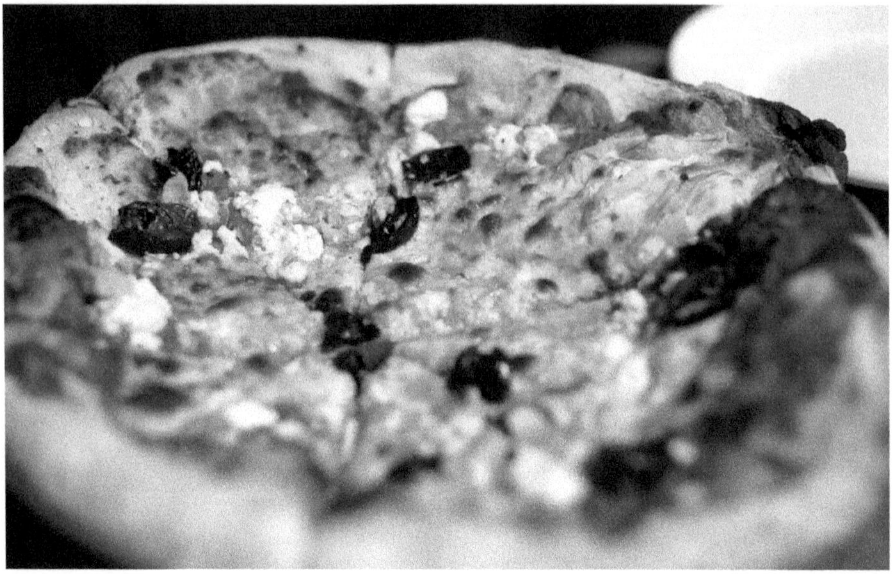

Preparation Time: 45 minutes.

Cooking Time: 35 minutes.

Servings: 3

Ingredients:

120 g tapioca flour

Teaspoon Celtic sea salt

1 tablespoon Italian spice mix

45 grams of coconut flour

120 ml olive oil (fresh) water (hot) 120 ml

Cover with eggs (slap):

1 tablespoon tomato paste (can)

1/2 slices zucchini

1/2 eggplant

Tomato slices
A spoon of olive oil (delicate)
Balsamic vinegar

Directions:

1. Preheat the oven to 190 ° C and cover the pan with parchment paper.

2. Cut the vegetables into thin slices.

3. Put cassava flour and salt, Italian herbs and coconut flour together in a large bowl.

4. Pour olive oil and hot water and mix well.

5. Then add the eggs and stir until the dough is even.

6. If it is too thin for the dough, add 1 tablespoon of coconut flour at a time until it reaches the desired thickness. Wait a few minutes before adding more coconut flour, as this will take some time to absorb the water. The purpose is to obtain a soft dough.

7. Divide the dough in half, then wrap it in a circle on the baking sheet (or make a large pizza as shown).

8. Bake for 10 minutes.

9. Brush the pizza with tomato sauce, then sprinkle the eggplant, zucchini and tomatoes on the pizza.

10. Pour the pancakes in olive oil and cook for 10 to15 minutes.
11. Pour balsamic vinegar on pizza before eating.

Nutrition: Calories:221.8 Fat:8.0 Carbs: 31g Protein: 12g

22. Vegetarian Ratatouille

Preparation Time: 20 minutes.

Cooking Time: 1 hour.

Servings: 1

Ingredients:

200 grams diced tomatoes (canned)

2 slices onion

Clove garlic

4 teaspoons dried oregano

4 c. 1 teaspoon paprika

A spoon of olive oil

Eggplant

Zucchini slices

Pepper

1 teaspoon dried thyme

Directions:

1. Preheat the oven to 180 ° C, then gently lubricate the circle or oval.

2. Finely chop onion and garlic.

3. Mix tomato slices with garlic, onion, oregano and pepper, season with salt and pepper, then put in the bottom of the pot.

4. Use a mandolin, cheese slicer or sharp knife to cut eggplant, zucchini and pepper.

5. Place the vegetables in a bowl (wrapped, starting at the edge and processing inside).

6. Place olive oil on vegetables and sprinkle with thyme, salt and pepper.

7. Cover the pan with parchment paper and bake for 45 to 55 minutes.

Nutrition: Calories: 130 Fat: 1g Carbs: 8g Protein:1g

23. Spicy Spare Ribs with Roasted Pumpkin

Preparation Time: 1 day.

Cooking Time: 1 hour and 15 minutes.

Servings: 5

Ingredients:

400g pork ribs

A spoon of coconut amino acids

Honey spoon

A spoon of olive oil

50 g shallots

Garlic clove

Green paper

1 slice onion

1 red pepper

1 red pepper

For the roasted pumpkin:

1 slice of pumpkin

1 tablespoon coconut oil

1 teaspoon of chili powder

Directions:

1. Pickled pork ribs the day before yesterday.

2. Cut the ribs into four small pieces: mix coconut amino acids, honey and olive oil in a bowl. Chopped green onions, garlic and peppers, then add.

Spread the ribs on the plastic container and pour the marinade. Place them in the refrigerator overnight.

3. Cut onions, peppers and peppers into small pieces and place in a slow cooker. Spare ribs (including marinade) and cook for at least 4 hours.

4. Preheat the pumpkin to 200 ° C.

5. Cut the pumpkin on the moon and place it on a baking sheet lined with parchment paper.

6. Place a spoonful of coconut oil on the baking sheet and season with chili, pepper and salt. Roast the pumpkin in the oven for about 20 minutes, and then serve with the ribs.

Nutrition: Calories: 282 Fat: 18g. Carbs:16g. Protein: 12g.

24. Roast Beef with Grilled Vegetables

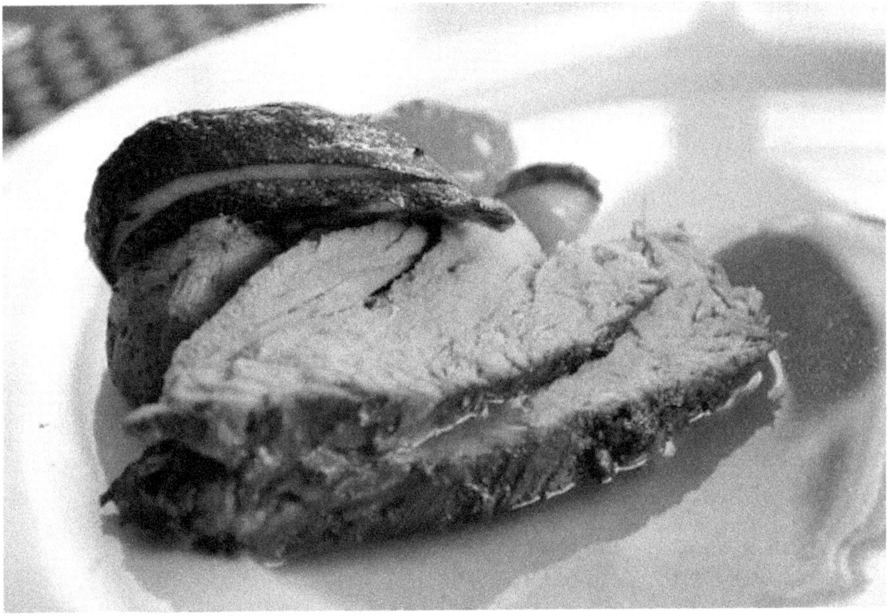

Preparation Time: 20 minutes.

Cooking Time: 1 hour and 10 minutes.

Servings: 5

Ingredients:

500 g roast beef

Garlic clove (squeezed)

One teaspoon fresh rosemary

400 g broccoli

200g carrots

400 g zucchini

A spoonful of olive oil

Directions:

1. Rub roast beef with sweet pepper, salt, garlic and rosemary.

2. Heat the pan over high heat and fry the meat for about 20 minutes, Or until, on all sides of the flesh, brown spots emerge.

3. Then wrap it with aluminum foil and let it sit for a while.

4. Before serving, slice the roast beef into thin slices.

5. Preheat the oven to 205 ° C. Put all the vegetables in the pan.

6. Season the vegetables with a little olive oil and then season with curry and paprika. Bake for 30 minutes or until the vegetables are cooked.

Nutrition: Calories: 347.6 Fat: 8.0g Carbs: 31g Protein: 32.2

25. Turkey meatball skewers

Preparation Time: 5 minutes
Cooking Time: 75 minutes
Servings: 4

Ingredients:
4 sticks of lemongrass
400g minced turkey
2 cloves of garlic, finely chopped
1 egg
1 red chili, finely chopped
2 tablespoons lime juice
2 tablespoons chopped coriander
1 teaspoon turmeric
Pepper

Directions:
1. Clean lemon grass cut in half lengthwise and wash.

2. Mix the meat with the egg, chili, garlic, coriander, olive oil, lime juice, turmeric and a little pepper. Make little balls out of them.

3. Put the balls on the lemongrass skewer and grill them as you like. Cook them in the oven or fry them in the pan until the balls are ready. A small salad goes with it.

Nutrition: Calories 280.0 Fat 35 g Cholesterol 340 mg Fiber 3 g Protein 2.6g

26. Avocado and Cannellini Mash Tacos

Preparation Time: 10 minutes

Ingredients:

1 ripe avocado, peeled and stoned

1 400g can of cannellini beans, drained Juice of 1/2 a lemon

1 table spoon olive oil

Salt and pepper

A couple of basil leaves

Taco shells

Directions:

Place the avocado into a bowl, approximately chop it and then mash it. Consist of the cannellini beans and lemon juice and mash them all together. Stir in the olive oil and season with salt and pepper. Destroy the basil leaves and consist of these.

Fill the taco shells and consume instantly!

27. Almond Butter and Alfalfa Wraps

Preparation Time: 10 minutes

Ingredients:

4 tablespoon of almond nut butter

Juice of 1 lemon

2-3 carrots-- grated

3 radishes, carefully sliced

1 cup of alfalfa sprouts

Salt and pepper

Lettuce leaves or nori sheets

Directions:

Mix the almond butter with the majority of the lemon juice and enough water to create a velvety consistency.

Combine the grated carrot, alfalfa sprouts in a bowl. Sprinkle with the remainder of the lemon juice and season with salt and pepper.

Spread the lettuce leaves or nori sheets with almond butter and top with the carrot and grow mixture. Roll up and consume instantly!

28. Asian King Prawn Stir-Fry with Buckwheat Noodles

Preparation time: 10 minutes
Cooking time: 15 minutes

Ingredients:

150g shelled raw king prawns, deveined
2 tea spoon tamari (you can use soy sauce if you are not avoiding gluten)
2 tea spoon extra virgin olive oil
75g soba (buckwheat noodles)
1 garlic clove, finely chopped
1 bird's eye chilli, finely chopped
1 tea spoon finely chopped fresh ginger
20g red onions, sliced
40g celery, trimmed and sliced
75g green beans, chopped
50g kale, roughly chopped
100ml chicken stock
5g lovage or celery leaves

Directions:

First heat a frying pan over a high first heat, then cook the prawns in 1 teaspoon of the tamari and 1 teaspoon of the oil for 2–3 minutes. Transfer the prawns to a plate. Wipe the pan out with kitchen paper, as you're going to use it again.

Cook the noodles in boiling water for 5–8 minutes or as directed on the packet. Drain and set aside.

Meanwhile, fry the garlic, chilli and ginger, red onion, celery, beans and kale in the remaining oil over a medium–high first heat for 2–3 minutes. Include the stock and bring to the boil, then simmer for a minute or two, until the vegetables are cooked but still crunchy. Include the prawns, noodles and lovage/celery leaves to the pan, bring back to the boil then remove from the first heat and dish out .

29. Savory Seed Truffles

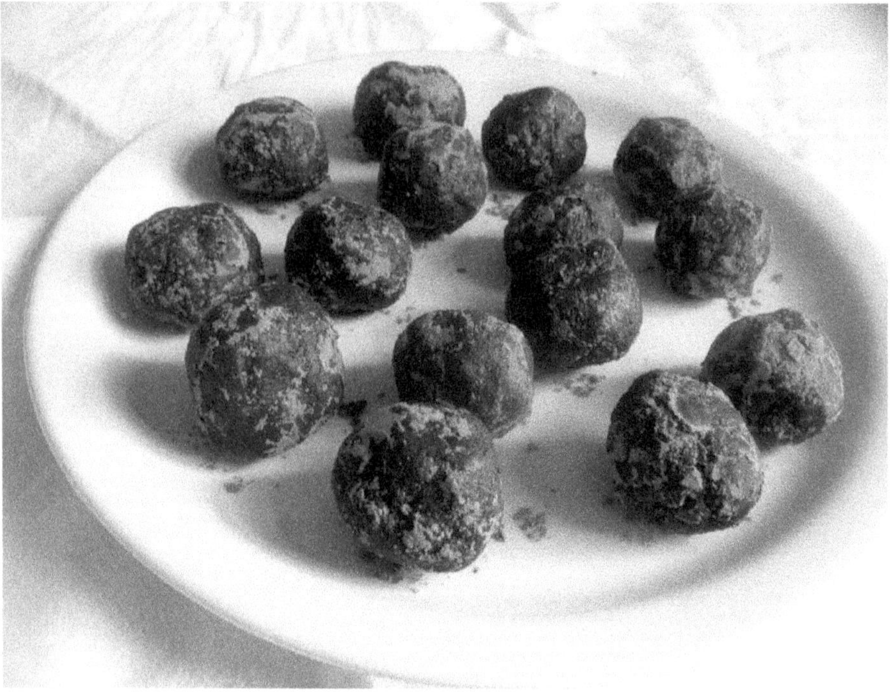

Preparation time: 10 minutes

Ingredients:

60g/2oz pumpkin seeds

60g/2oz sunflower seeds

2 table spoon tahini

Pinch of cayenne pepper

Juice of half a lemon

A handful of coriander leaves

Salt and pepper

Directions:

Place the seeds in a food mill with the S blade and grind thoroughly. Include the tahini, cayenne, lemon juice, coriander leaves and salt and pepper.

Process till the mix holds together includeing little quantities of water as r eq uired.

Get rid of the blade from the food mill and form the mix into walnut sized balls.

30. Turmeric Chicken & Kale Salad with Honey Lime Dressing

Preparation time: 20 minutes
Cooking time: 10 minutes

Ingredients:

For the chicken
1 teaspoon ghee or 1 table spoon coconut oil ½ medium brown onion, diced
250-300 g / 9 oz. chicken mince or diced up chicken thighs
1 large garlic clove, finely diced
1 teaspoon turmeric powder
1teaspoon lime zest
juice of ½ lime
½ teaspoon salt + pepper

For the salad
6 broccolini stalks or 2 cups of broccoli florets
2 tablespoons pumpkin seeds (pepitas)
3 large kale leaves, stems removed and chopped
½ avocado, sliced
handful of fresh coriander leaves, chopped handful of fresh parsley leaves, chopped
For the dressing
3 tablespoons lime juice
1 small garlic clove, finely diced or grated
3 tablespoons extra-virgin olive oil (I used 1 tablespoons avocado oil and * 2 tablespoons
EVO)

1 teaspoon raw honey

½ teaspoon wholegrain or Dijon mustard

½ teaspoon sea salt and pepper

Directions:

1. First heat the ghee or coconut oil in a small frying pan over medium-high first heat. Include the onion and sauté on medium first heat for 4-5 minutes, until golden. Include the chicken mince and garlic and stir for 2-3 minutes over medium-high first heat, breaking it apart.

2. Include the turmeric, lime zest, lime juice, salt and pepper and cook, stirring frequently, for a further 3-4 minutes. Set the cooked mince aside.

3. While the chicken is cooking, bring a small saucepan of water to boil. Include the broccolini and cook for 2 minutes. Rinse under cold water and cut into 3-4 pieces each.

4. Include the pumpkin seeds to the frying pan from the chicken and toast over medium first heat for 2 minutes, stirring fr eq uently to prevent burning. Season with a little salt. Set aside. Raw pumpkin seeds are also fine to use.

5. Place chopped kale in a salad bowl and pour over the dressing. Using your hands, toss and
massage the kale with the dressing. This will soften the kale, kind of like what citrus juice does to fish or beef carpaccio – it 'cooks' it slightly.

6. Finally toss through the cooked chicken, broccolini, fresh herbs, pumpkin seeds and avocado
slices.

31. Moong Dahl

ù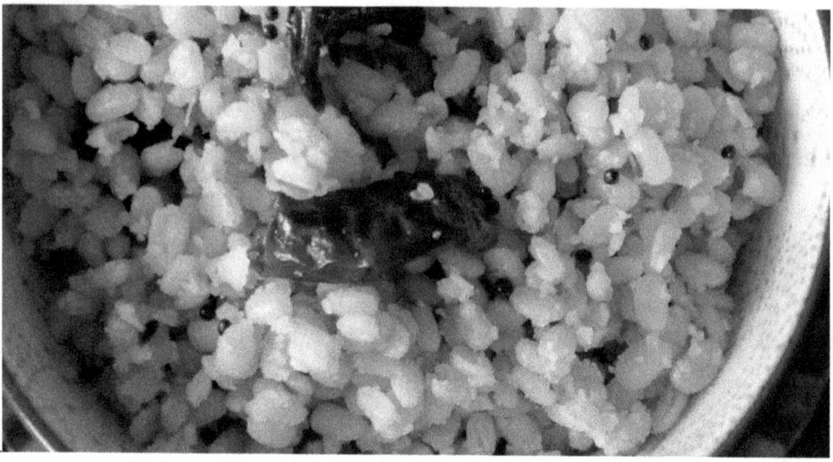

Preparation time: 10 minutes

Cooking time: 15 minutes

Ingredients:

300g/10oz split mung beans (moong dahl)-- preferably soaked for a couple of hours

600ml/1pt of water

2 table spoon/30g olive butter, oil or ghee

1 red onion, finely chopped

1-2 tea spoon coriander seeds

1-2 tea spoon cumin seeds

2-4 tea spoon fresh ginger, sliced

1-2 tea spoon turmeric

If you desire it spicy, 1/4 tea spoon of cayenne pepper--more.

Salt & black pepper to taste.

Directions:

Drain and wash the split mung beans. Put them in a pan and cover with the water. Give the boil and skim off any foam that occurs. Decline the very first heat, cover and simmer.

First heat the oil in a pan and sauté the onion till soft.

Dry fry the coriander and cumin seeds in a heavy bottomed pan up until they start to pop. Grind them in a pestle and mortar.

Consist of the ground spices to the onions in addition to the cayenne, turmeric and ginger pepper. Cook for a few minutes.

When the mung beans are almost cooked include the onion and spice mix to them. Season with salt and pepper and cook for an additional 10 minutes.

32. Buckwheat Noodles with Chicken Kale & Miso Dressing

Preparation time: 10 minutes

Cooking time: 15 minutes

Ingredients:

For the noodles

2-3 handfuls of kale leaves (removed from the stem and roughly cut)

150 g / 5 oz buckwheat noodles (100% buckwheat, no wfirst heat)

3-4 shiitake mushrooms, sliced

1 teaspoon coconut oil or ghee

1 brown onion, finely diced

1 medium free-range chicken breast, sliced or diced

1 long red chilli, thinly sliced (seeds in or out depending on how hot you like it)

2 large garlic cloves, finely diced

2-3 tablespoons Tamari sauce (gluten-free soy sauce)

For the miso dressing

1½ tablespoon fresh organic miso

1 tablespoon Tamari sauce

1 tablespoon extra-virgin olive oil

1 tablespoon lemon or lime juice

1 teaspoon sesame oil (optional)

Directions:

1. Bring a medium saucepan of water to boil. Include the kale and cook for 1 minute, until

slightly wilted. Remove and set aside but reserve the water and bring it back to the boil. Include the soba noodles and cook according to the package steps (usually about 5 minutes). Rinse under cold water and set aside.

2. In the meantime, pan fry the shiitake mushrooms in a little ghee or coconut oil (about a teaspoon) for 2-3 minutes, until lightly browned on each side. Sprinkle with
sea salt and set aside.

3. In the same frying pan, first heat more coconut oil or ghee over medium-high first heat. Sauté onion and chilli for 2-3 minutes and then include the chicken pieces. Cook 5 minutes over medium first heat, stirring a couple of times, then include the garlic, tamari sauce and a little splash of water. Cook for a further 2-3 minutes, stirring fr eq uently until chicken is cooked through.

4. Finally, include the kale and soba noodles and toss through the chicken to warm up.

5. Mix the miso dressing and drizzle over the noodles right at the end of cooking, this way you will keep all those beneficial probiotics in the miso alive and active.

33. Courgette Tortilla

Preparation time: 10 minutes

Cooking time: 15 minutes

Ingredients:

2 table spoon coconut oil or butter

1 courgettes, sliced

4 eggs, beaten

A pinch of salt and pepper

Newly chopped chives or parsley

Directions:

First heat the oil or butter in a heavy bottomed fry pan and consist of the courgettes. Prepare until soft, stirring sometimes.

Mix the salt, pepper, and herbs in with the beaten eggs and consist of to the pan.

Cook till the egg is almost cooked through. End up the cooking by positioning the pan under a medium grill. Dish out with a large green salad.

34. Baked Potatoes with Spicy Chickpea Stew

Preparation time: 10 minutes

Cooking time: 45 minutes

Ingredients:

4-6 baking potatoes, punctured all over

2 tablespoons olive oil

2 red onions, finely sliced

4 cloves garlic, grated or crushed

2cm ginger, grated

1/2 -2 teaspoons chilli flakes (depending on how hot you like things)

2 tablespoons cumin seeds

2 tablespoons turmeric

Splash of water

2 x 400g tins sliced tomatoes

2 tablespoons unsweetened cocoa powder (or cacao)

If you prefer) consisting of the chickpea water DON'T DRAIN!!

2 yellow peppers (or whatever colour you prefer!), 2 x 400g tins chickpeas (or kidney beans,sliced into bitesize pieces

2 tablespoons parsley plus additional for garnish Salt and pepper to taste (optional) Side salad (optional)

Directions:

Prefirst heat the microwave to 400F, meanwhile you can prepare all your things required. When the microwave is hot sufficient location your baking potatoes in the microwave and cook for 1 hour or until they are done how you like them. When the potatoes are in the microwave, position the olive oil and chopped red onion in a big broad pan and cook carefully, with the lid on for 5 minutes, till the onions are not brown however soft. Remove the cover and include the garlic, chilli, ginger and cumin. Cook for a more minute on a low first heat, then consist of the turmeric and a really small splash of water and cook for another minute, taking care not to let the pan get too dry. Next, include in the tomatoes, cocoa powder (or cacao), chickpeas (consisting of the chickpea water) and yellow pepper. Bring to the boil, then simmer on a low very first heat for 45 minutes till the sauce is thick and unctuous (but do not let it burn!). The stew must be done at roughly the same time as the potatoes. Stir in the 2 tablespoons of parsley, and some salt and pepper if you wish, and meal out the stew on top of the baked potatoes, maybe with a basic side salad.

35. Fragrant Asian Hotpot

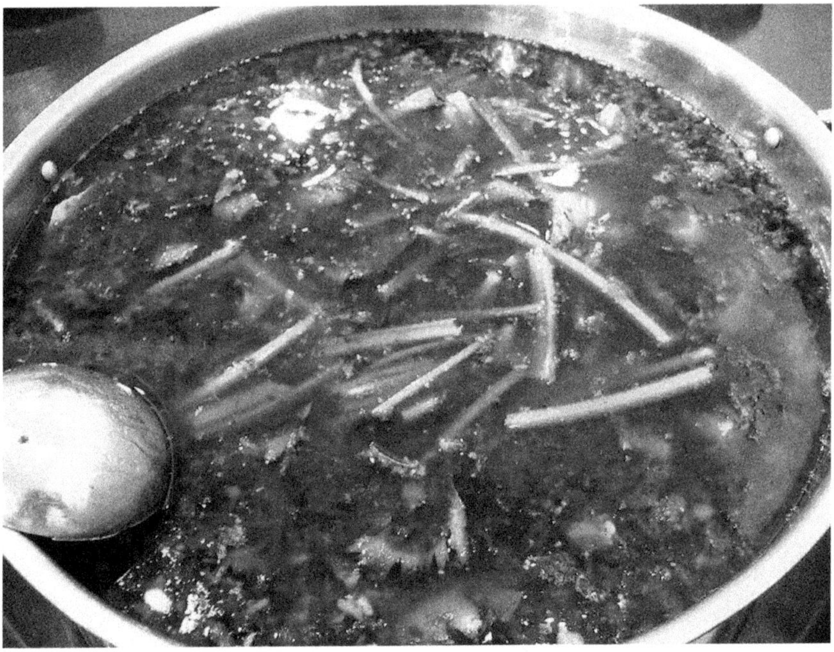

Preparation time: 10 minutes

Cooking time: 10 minutes

Ingredients:

1 tea spoon tomato purée

1 star anise, crushed (or 1/4 tea spoon ground anise) Small handful (10g) parsley, stalks carefully chopped Little handful (1Og) coriander, stalks finely sliced Juice of 1/2 lime.

500ml chicken stock, fresh or made with 1 cube 1/2 carrot, peeled and cut into matchsticks 50g broccoli, cut into little florets 50g beansprouts

100 g raw tiger prawns

100 g company tofu, sliced

50g rice noodles, prepared according to packet actions
50g prepared water chestnuts, drained pipes
20g sushi ginger, chopped
1 table spoon good-quality miso paste

Directions:

Location the tomato purée, star anise, parsley stalks, coriander stalks, lime juice and chicken

stock in a big pan and bring to a simmer for 10 minutes. Consist of the carrot, broccoli, prawns, tofu, noodles and water chestnuts and simmer gently up until the prawns are cooked through. Get rid of from the first heat and stir in the sushi ginger and miso paste.

Dispense sprinkled with the parsley and coriander leaves.

36. Chargrilled Beef With A Red Wine Jus, Onion Rings, Garlic Kale And Herb Roasted Potatoes

Preparation time: 10 minutes

Cooking time: 50 minutes

Ingredients:

100g potatoes, peeled and cut into 2cm dice

1 table spoon extra virgin olive oil

5g parsley, carefully sliced

50g red onion, sliced into rings

50g kale, sliced

1 garlic clove, carefully chopped

120-- 150g x 3.5cm-thick beef fillet steak or 2cm-thick sirloin steak

40ml red white wine

150ml beef stock

1 tea spoon tomato purée

1 tea spoon cornflour, liquified in 1 table spoon water

Directions:

First heat the microwave to 440F/ gas 7.

Location the potatoes in a saucepan of boiling water, bring back to the boil and cook for 4-- 5 minutes, then drain. Location in a roasting tin with 1 teaspoon of the oil and roast in the hot microwave oven for 35-- 45 minutes.

Fry the onion in 1 teaspoon of the oil over a medium first heat for 5-- 7 minutes, until soft and well caramelised. Fry the garlic gently in 1/2 teaspoon of oil for 1 minute, up until soft but not coloured. Include the kale and fry for a further 1-- 2 minutes, till tender. First heat an microwave ovenproof fry pan over a high first heat up until smoking cigarettes.

Cover the meat in 1/2 a teaspoon of the oil and fry in the hot pan over a medium-- high first heat according to how you like your meat done.If you like your meat medium it would be better to sear the meat and then move the pan to a microwave set at 440F/ gas 7 and finish the cooking that method for the prescribed times. Eliminate the meat from the pan and set aside to rest. Consist of the red wine to the hot pan to bring up any meat residue. Bubble to decrease the red wine by half, until syrupy and with a concentrated taste. Consist of the stock and tomato purée to the steak pan and give the boil, then include the cornflour paste to thicken your sauce, including it a little at a time until you have your desired consistency. Stir in any of the juices from the rested steak and dispense with the roasted potatoes, kale, onion rings and red wine sauce.

37. Kale, Edamame, and Tofu Curry

Preparation time: 10 minutes

Cooking time: 50 minutes

Ingredients:

1 table spoon rapeseed oil

1 big onion, chopped

4 cloves garlic, peeled and grated

1 large thumb (7cm) fresh ginger, peeled and grated

1 red chilli, deseeded and thinly sliced

1/2 tea spoon ground turmeric

1/4 tea spoon cayenne pepper

1 tea spoon paprika

1/2 tea spoon ground cumin

1 tea spoon salt

250g dried red lentils

1 litre boiling water

50g frozen soya edamame beans

200g company tofu, chopped into cubes 2 tomatoes, approximately sliced

Juice of 1 lime

200g kale leaves, stalks eliminated and torn

Directions:

Include the onion and cook for 5 minutes prior to including the garlic, chilli and ginger and

cooking for a further 2 minutes. Stir through before including the red lentils and stirring once again.

Put in the boiling water and bring to a hearty simmer for 10 minutes, then minimize the very first heat and cook for a further 20-30 minutes till the curry has a thick '- porridge' consistency.

Consist of the soya beans, tofu and tomatoes and cook for a further 5 minutes. Consist of the lime juice and kale leaves and cook until the kale is simply tender.

38. Sirtfood Mushroom Scramble Eggs

Preparation time: 10 minutes
Cooking time: 10 minutes

Ingredients:

2 eggs.
1 tea spoon ground turmeric
1 teaspoon mild curry powder
20g kale, roughly sliced
1 tea spoon additional virgin olive oil
1/2 bird's eye chilli, very finely sliced
handful of button mushrooms, very finely sliced 5g parsley, carefully chopped optional Include a seed mixture as a topper and some Rooster Sauce for taste.

Directions:

Mix the turmeric and curry powder and consist of a little water until you have achieved a light paste.
Steam the kale for 2-- 3 minutes.
Heat the oil in a frying pan over a medium very first heat and fry the chilli and mushrooms for 2-- 3 minutes up until they have actually begun to brown and soften.

39. Fragrant Chicken Breast with Kale, Red Onion, and Salsa-Sirtfood

Preparation time: 10 minutes

Cooking time: 15 minutes

Ingredients:

120g skinless, boneless chicken breast

2 tea spoon ground turmeric

juice of 1/4 lemon

1 table spoon additional virgin olive oil

50g kale, chopped.

20g red onion, sliced

1 tea spoon chopped fresh ginger

50g buckwheat

Directions:

To make the salsa, remove the eye from the tomato and slice it really finely, taking care to keep as much of the l iq uid as possible. Blend with the chilli, capers, parsley and lemon juice. You might put everything in the end however a blender outcome is a bit different. First heat the microwave oven to 440F/ gas 7. Marinate the chicken breast in 1 teaspoon of the turmeric, a little oil and the lemon juice. Leave for 5-- 10 minutes.

Very first heat an microwave ovenproof frying pan until hot, then include the marinated chicken and cook for a minute approximately on each side, up until pale golden, then transfer to the microwave (put on a baking tray if your pan isn't microwave ovenproof) for 8-- 10 minutes or till prepared through. Eliminate from the microwave, cover with foil and leave to rest for 5 minutes before serving.

Prepare the kale in a steamer for 5 minutes. Fry the red onions and the ginger in a little oil, up until soft however not coloured, then consist of the prepared kale and fry for another minute. Cook the buckwheat according to the packet actions with the staying teaspoon of turmeric. Dish outalongside the chicken, vegetables and salsa.

40. Smoked Salmon Omelette

Preparation time: 10 minutes

Cooking time: 10 minutes

Ingredients:

2 Medium eggs

100 g Smoked salmon, sliced

1/2 tea spoon Capers

10 g Rocket, chopped

1 teaspoon Parsley, sliced

1 tea spoon Extra virgin olive oil

Directions:

Split the eggs into a bowl and blend well. Include the salmon, capers, rocket and parsley.

Very first heat the olive oil in a non-stick fry pan up until hot however not cigarette smoking.

Consist of the egg mix and, using a spatula or fish piece, move the mix around the pan until it is even. Reduce the first heat and let the omelette cook through. Slide the spatula around the edges and roll up or fold the omelette in half to dispense.

41. Sirt Food Miso Marinated Cod with Stir-Fried Greens & Sesame

Preparation time: 10 minutes
Cooking time: 15 minutes

Ingredients:

20g miso
1 table spoon mirin
1 tablespoon extra virgin olive oil
200g skinless cod fillet
20g red onion, sliced
40g celery, sliced
1 garlic clove, finely sliced
1 bird's eye chilli, finely sliced
1 tea spoon finely chopped fresh ginger
60g green beans
50g kale, approximately sliced
1 tea spoon sesame seeds
5g parsley, roughly chopped
1 table spoon tamari
30g buckwheat
1 tea spoon ground turmeric

Directions:

Mix the miso, mirin and 1 teaspoon of the oil. Rub all over the cod and delegate marinate for 30 minutes. Heat the microwave oven to 440F/ gas 7. Bake the cod for 10 minutes.

Include the onion and stir-fry for a few minutes, then consist of the celery, garlic, chilli, ginger, green beans and kale. You might require to consist of a little water to the pan

to help the cooking process. Prepare the buckwheat according to the packet steps with the turmeric for 3 minutes. Consist of the sesame seeds, parsley and tamari to the stir-fry and meal outwith the greens and fish.

42. Vietnamese Turmeric Fish with Herbs & Mango Sauce-New

Preparation time: 15 minutes
Cooking time: 30 minutes

Ingredients:
Fish:
1 1/4 pounds fresh cod boneless, skinless and fish, cut into 2-inch piece large that have to do
with 1/2 inch thick
If essential), * 2 table spoon coconut oil to pan-fry the fish (plus a couple of more tablespoon
Small pinch of sea salt to taste
Fish marinade: (Marinate for at least 1 hr. or as long as overnight)
1 table spoon turmeric powder
1 teaspoon sea salt
1 table spoon Chinese cooking red wine (Alt. dry sherry)
2 tea spoon minced ginger
2 table spoon olive oil
Instilled Scallion and Dill Oil:
2 cups scallions (piece into long thin shape)
2 cups of fresh dill
Pinch of sea salt to taste
Mango dipping sauce:
1 medium sized ripe mango
2 table spoon rice vinegar
Juice of 1/2 lime
1 garlic clove
1 tea spoon dry red chili pepper (stir in prior to serving)

Toppings:
Fresh cilantro (as much as you like)
Lime juice (as much as you like)
Nuts (cashew or pine nuts)

Directions:

1. Marinade the fish for a minimum of 1 hr. or as long as over night.

2. Location all things r eq uired under "Mango Dipping Sauce" into a food mill and blend till
wanted consistency.

To Pan-Fry The Fish:
First heat 2 table spoon of coconut oil in a non-stick big frying pan over high very first heat.
When hot, consist of the pre-marinated fish. * Note: place the fish slices into the pan individually and separate to two or more batches to pan fry if essential. You should hear a loud sizzle, after which you can reduce the very first heat to medium-high. Do not move the fish or turn up until you see a golden brown color on the side, about 5 minutes.
Season with a pinch of sea salt. Consist of of more coconut oil to pan-fry the fish is essential.* Note: There need to be some oil left in the frying pan. We utilize the remainder of the oil to make scallion and dill instilled oil.
To Make The Scallion And Dill Infused Oil:.
Utilize the rest of the oil in the fry pan over medium-high first heat, include 2 cups of scallions and 2 cups of dill. Once you have actually includeed the scallions and dill, turn off the first heat.
Provide a gentle toss just up until the scallions and dill have actually wilted, about 15 seconds. Season with a dash of sea salt.
Pour the scallion, dill, and instilled oil over the fish and dish outwith mango dipping sauce with fresh cilantro, lime, and nuts.

43. Moroccan Spiced Eggs

Preparation time: 10 minutes

Cooking time: 15 minutes

Ingredients:

1 tea spoon olive oil

1 shallot, peeled and finely chopped

1 red (bell) pepper, deseeded and finely sliced

1 garlic clove, peeled and carefully chopped

1 courgette (zucchini), peeled and finely chopped

1 table spoon tomato puree (paste)

1/2 tea spoon mild chilli powder

1/4 tea spoon ground cinnamon

1/4 tea spoon ground cumin

1/2 tea spoon salt

1 × 400g (14oz) can sliced tomatoes.

1 x 400g (14oz) can chickpeas in water.

small handful of flat-leaf parsley (10g (1/3oz)), sliced.

4 medium eggs at room temperature.

Directions:

- First heat the oil in a saucepan, include the shallot and red (bell) pepper and fry carefully for 5 minutes. Include the garlic and courgette (zucchini) and cook for another minute or two. Consist of the tomato puree (paste), spices and salt and stir through.

- Include the chopped tomatoes and chickpeas (soaking alcohol and all) and increase the very first heat to medium. With the cover off the pan, simmer the sauce for 30 minutes-- make sure it is gently bubbling throughout and permit it to minimize in volume by about one-third.

- Remove from the very first heat and stir in the chopped parsley.

- Prefirst heat the microwave oven to 200C/180C fan/350F.

- When you are prepared to cook the eggs, bring the tomato sauce as much as a gentle simmer and transfer to a little microwave oven-proof meal.

- Crack the eggs on the side of the meal and lower them gently into the stew. Cover with foil and bake in the microwave oven for 10-15 minutes. Meal outthe concoction in individual bowls with the eggs drifting on the top.

44. Savory Sirtfood Salmon

Ingredients:

Salmon, 5 oz

Lemon juice, 1 tbsp

Ground turmeric, 1 tsp

Extra virgin olive oil, 2 tbsp

1 chopped red onion

1 finely chopped garlic clove

1 finely chopped bird's eye chili

Quinoa, 2 oz

Finely chopped ginger, fresh, 1 tsp

Celery, chopped, 1 cup

Parsley, chopped, 1 tbsp

Tomato, diced, 4.5 oz

Vegetable stock, 100 ml

Directions:

Preheat your oven to 200 °C. Fry the celery, chili, garlic, onion, and ginger on olive oil up to three minutes. Add quinoa, tomatoes, and the chicken stock and let simmer for another ten minutes. Layer olive oil, lemon juice, and turmeric on top of the salmon and bake for ten minutes. Add parsley and celery before serving.

45. Sirtfood Miso Salmon

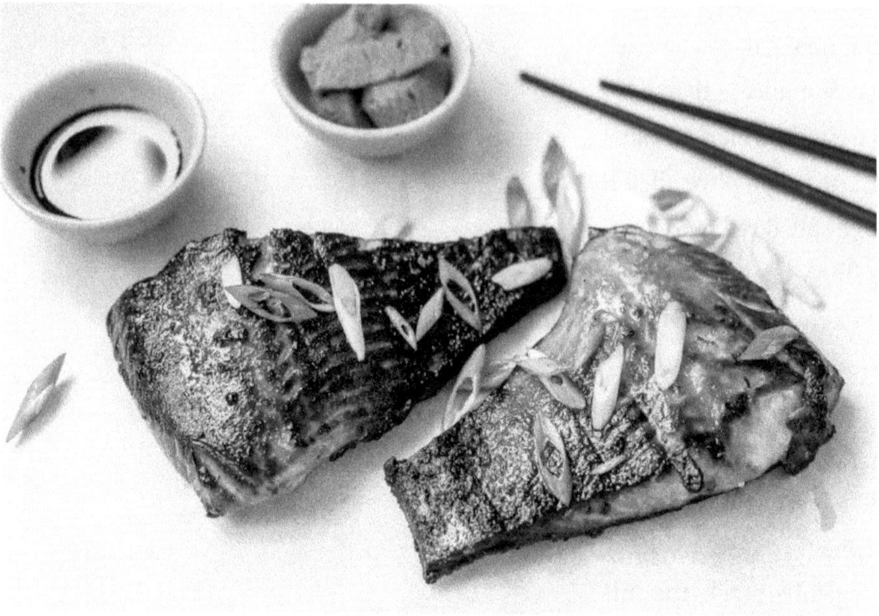

Planning time: 15 min.

Cooking time: 30 min.

Servings: 4

Ingredients:

Miso, ½ cup

Organic red wine, 1 tbsp

Extra virgin olive oil, 1 tbsp

Salmon, 7 oz

1 sliced red onion

Celery, sliced, 1 cup

2 finely chopped garlic cloves

1 finely chopped bird's eye chili

Ground turmeric, 1 tsp

Freshly chopped ginger, 1 tsp

Green beans, 1 cup

Kale, finely chopped, 1 cup

Sesame seeds. 1 tsp

Soy sauce, 1 tbsp

Buckwheat, 2 tbsp

Directions:

Marinate the salmon in the mix of red wine, 1 tsp of extra virgin olive oil, and miso for 30 minutes. Preheat the oven to 420 °F and bake for 10 minutes with the cod.

Fry the onions, chili, garlic, green beans, ginger, kale, and celery for a few minutes until it's cooked. Insert the soy sauce, parsley, and sesame seeds. Cook buckwheat per instructions and mix in with the stir-fry.

46. Sirtfood Salmon with Kale Salad

Planning time: 15 min.

Cooking time: 18 min.

Servings: 4

Ingredients:

Salmon, 4 oz

2 sliced red onions

Parsley, chopped, 1 oz

Cucumber, 2 oz

2 sliced radishes

Spinach, ½ cup

Salad leaves, ½ cup

Salad dressing

Raw honey, 1 tsp

Greek yogurt, 1 tbsp

Lemon juice, 1 tbsp

Chopped mint leaves, 2 tbsp

A pinch of salt

A pinch of pepper

Directions:

Preheat your oven to 200 °C. Bake the salmon for up to 18 minutes and set aside. Mix in the ingredients for dressing and leave to sit between five and ten minutes.

Serve the salad with spinach and top with parsley, onions, cucumber, and radishes.

47. Spicy Sirtfood Ricotta

Ingredients:

Extra virgin olive oil, 2 tsp

Unsalted ricotta cheese, 200 g

Pinch of salt

Pinch of pepper

1 chopped red onion

1 tsp of fresh ginger

1 finely sliced garlic clove

1 finely sliced green chili

1 cup diced cherry tomatoes

½ tsp ground cumin

½ tsp ground coriander

½ tsp mild chili powder Chopped parsley, ½ cup Fresh spinach leaves, 2 cup

Directions:

Heat olive oil in a lidded pan over high heat. Toss in the ricotta cheese, seasoning it with pepper and sea salt. Fry until it turns golden and removes it from the pan. Add the onion to the pan and reduce the heat. Fry the onion with chili, ginger, and garlic for around eight minutes and add the chopped tomatoes. Using the lid to cover and cook for another five minutes.

Add the remaining spices and sea salt to the cheese, put the cheese back into the pan and stir, adding spinach, coriander, and parsley. Use the lid to cover and cook for another two minutes.

48. Vietnamese Turmeric Fish with Herbs & Mango Sauce

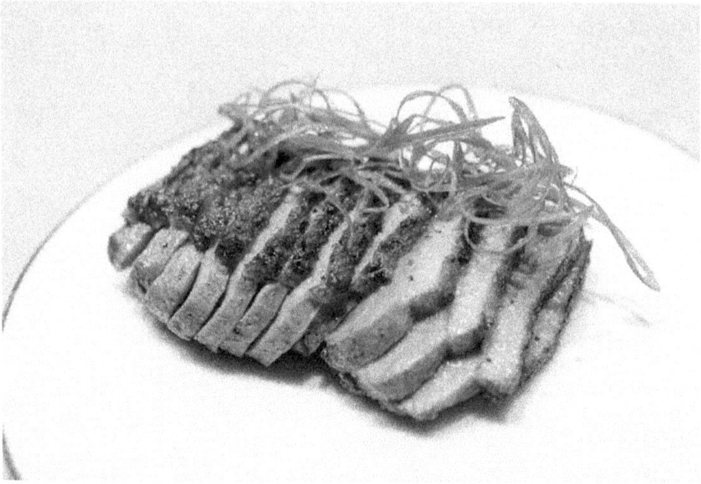

Ingredients:

Fish:

Fresh codfish, boneless one ¼ lb

coconut oil 2 tbsp

A little pinch of sea salt

Marinading fish: (Marinate for at least 1 hr. or as long as overnight)

Turmeric powder 1 tbsp

Sea salt 1 tsp

Chinese cooking wine 1 tbsp

Minced ginger 2 tsp

Olive oil 2 tbsp

Infused Scallion and Dill Oil:

Scallions 2 cups

Dill 2 cups of fresh

Pinch of sea salt

Mango dipping sauce:
Ripe mango one medium-sized
Rice vinegar 2 tbsp
Juice of ½ lime
Garlic one clove
Dry red chili pepper 1 tsp

Directions:

1. Marinate the fish for at least 1 hour or overnight for as long as practicable.

2. Put all ingredients in a food processor under "Mango Dipping Sauce" and blend until consistency is desired.

To the Fish Pan-Fry:

1. In a big, non-stick frying pan over high heat, heat 2 tbsp of coconut oil. Then add the pre-marinated fish when heated. * Note: put the fish slices separately in the pan and if appropriate, divide them into two or three batches to pan fry.

2. A noisy sizzle can be detected, during which you should reduce the medium-high heat.

3. Don't switch or move the fish for around 5 minutes before seeing the golden-brown color on foot. Using a touch of sea salt to season. To pan-fry the fish, if appropriate, add more coconut oil.

4. When the fish is golden brown, gently move the fish to the other side to cook. Move it to a wide plate until it's finished. *Note: The frying pan may

have some oil remaining. To render scallion and dill flavored oil, we use the remainder of the oil.

To make the Flavored Oil Scallion and Dill:

1. Using most of the oil over medium-high heat in the frying pan, then apply 2 cups of scallions and 2 cups of dill. Once you have the scallions and dill attached, switching off the heat, offer them a soft toss for around 15 seconds, only before the scallions and dill have wilted. Season with a dash of salt from the sea.

2. Pour over the fish with the scallion, dill, and flavored oil and serve with new cilantro, lime, and nuts with mango dipping sauce.

49. Sirtfood Chicken Breasts

Prep Time: 15 mins

Cook Time: 15 mins

Ingredients:

120 g skinless, boneless chicken breast Two tsp. ground Tumeric juice of 1/4 lemon One tbsp. extra virgin olive oil

50 g kale, chopped

Twenty g red onion, chopped

One tsp. fresh ginger

50 g buckwheat

For the Salsa:

130 g tomato

One bird's eye chili, finely chopped

One tbsp. capers, finely chopped

Five g parsley, finely chopped juice of 1/4 lemon

Directions:

To make the salsa, remove the eye

from the tomato and chop it very thinly, taking care to retain as much of the liquid as possible. Chili, capers, parsley, and lemon juice are mixed together. You could put it all in a blender, but the end result is a little different.

Heat the furnace to 220oC/gas 7. Using 1 teaspoon of turmeric, lemon juice, and a little oil to marinate the chicken breast. Leave yourself for 5-10 minutes.

Heat the ovenproof frying pan until hot, then add the marinated chicken and cook until pale golden on each side for about a minute, then transfer to the oven for 8-10 minutes or until cooked through (place on a baking tray if your pan is not ovenproof). Remove from the oven, cover with foil, and leave for 5 minutes to rest before serving.

Meanwhile, cook the kale for 5 minutes in a steamer. In a little oil, fry the red onions and the ginger until soft but not colored, then stir in the cooked kale and fry for another minute.

Cook the buckwheat with the remaining teaspoon of turmeric according to the packet directions. Serve alongside the salsa, tomatoes, and chicken.

50. Sweet-Smelling Chicken Breast, Kale, Red Onion, and Salsa

Planning time: 55 min

Cooking time: 30 min

Servings: 2

Ingredients:

120g skinless, boneless chicken bosom 2 teaspoons ground turmeric

20g red onion, cut

1 teaspoon new ginger, sliced 50g buckwheat ¼ lemon

1 tablespoon extra-virgin olive oil 50 g kale, cleaved

Directions:

To set up the salsa, remove the tomato eye and finely cut. Include the chili, parsley, capers, lemon juice, and blend.

Preheat the oven to 220°C. Pour 1 teaspoon of the turmeric, the lemon juice, and a little oil on the chicken bosom and marinate. Permit to remain for 5–10 minutes.

Place an ovenproof griddle on the warmth and cook the marinated chicken for a moment on each side to accomplish a pale brilliant color. At that point move the container containing the chicken to the oven and permit to remain for 8–10 minutes or until it is finished. Remove from the oven and spread with foil, put in a safe place for 5 minutes before serving.

Put the kale in a liner and cook for 5 minutes. Pour a little oil in a pan and fry the red onions and the ginger to turn out to be delicate yet not shaded. Include the cooked kale and keep on frying for another minute.

Cook the buckwheat adhering to the bundle's guidelines utilizing the rest of the turmeric. Serve close by the chicken, salsa, and vegetables.